Physical Education Reinvented

Active and Collaborative Learning

Table of Contents

Chapter 1. Introduction

Get ready to plunge into the vibrant world of Physical Education unlike any other! In our Special Report "Physical Education Reinvented: Active and Collaborative Learning," we're turning the conventional wisdom on its head. No more will gym class mean droning hours of running laps and performing rote drills. We're bringing you a fresh, exciting perspective that taps into the joy of sports, the spirit of teamwork, and the thrill of personal development. This isn't just any rebranding; it's a revolution, redefining how we perceive fitness training and a revolution to make every kid look forward to PE class. Empowering, enlightening, and enlivening - this is a report that's certain to make you see Physical Education in a completely new light. Your journey towards changing lives starts here, one active, engaged, and enthusiastic learner at a time! Secure your copy of our Special Report now and be part of this transformative movement!

Chapter 2. Laying the Groundwork: The New Paradigm in Physical Education

Physical Education (PE) has traditionally been viewed as an ancillary aspect of the educational experience - a time to let students burn off some steam and get some exercise, but not as a vital piece of their academic journey. This misconception has done a disservice to students and to the educational community. PE allows students to grasp important life skills promoting teamwork, determination, and resilience. It has profound impact on cognitive development, instills a love for fitness, and also provides a platform for teaching social skills.

2.1. Shifting The Perspective

The new paradigm in Physical Education marks a dramatic shift away from the traditional PE model. This game-changing approach seeks to genuinely engage students in a way that fosters enthusiasm, positivity, and commitment to fitness. The new paradigm positions PE as an enjoyable, cooperative, inspiring, and indispensable part of the curriculum, making it something students eagerly anticipate.

The groundbreaking principle of this paradigm is the recognition that every child is unique, harboring different interests, strengths, and challenges, and education must honor this individuality. Instead of focusing solely on competitive sports and rigorous exercise, the new paradigm focuses on broadening PE to include activities that promote lifelong fitness habits, teamwork, and individual growth.

2.2. The Context of the New Paradigm

A significant insight of this new paradigm is that for learning to be truly effective, it must be relevant to the student's context. The new PE model emphasizes activities that relate directly to the students' day-to-day lives and can blend seamlessly with their routines.

In this paradigm, climbing a rope, a common PE exercise, goes beyond mere physical exertion, rope climbing metamorphoses into an allegory for overcoming personal challenges, exhibiting determination, and celebrating progress. This wider context turns a mundane exercise into a rich learning experience.

2.3. Focus on Collaboration

Competitive sports undeniably teach students valuable lessons about life. Yet, there's a pressing need to reposition the role of competition in PE. By allowing cooperative and team-building activities to take center stage, PE encourages students to celebrate not only their own successes but also those of their classmates.

Collaborative strategies such as group fitness challenges, paired exercises, and cooperative games not only boost the overall fitness level but also instill an appreciation for team dynamics and collective victories.

2.4. Cultivating Inclusivity

A cornerstone of this new paradigm is ensuring inclusion. Regardless of their physical abilities, every child has the right to fully participate in physical education. To this end, we need to devise activities that accommodate all levels of abilities.

This may involve adapting traditional games, introducing assistive technologies, or utilizing an individualized approach for some students. The goal is to provide an encouraging learning environment where every student feels comfortable.

2.5. Personal Development and Emotional Well-being

The psychological benefits of physical activity are now widely recognized. The new PE model puts emphasis on promoting emotional well-being, resilience, and stress management skills, alongside physical fitness.

Mindfulness and relaxation techniques, yoga, and tai chi, besides the usual sports activities, are incorporated into the teaching methodology. These practices strengthen the mind-body connection and foster mental well-being.

2.6. Technology Integration

Technology promises an innovative way to motivate students, improve performance, and track improvements. Using wearables to monitor heart rate, apps to track physical activity, or virtual reality to introduce students to new sports, the combination of PE and technology can revolutionize the learning process.

In the end, the goal of this new paradigm in Physical Education is to turn the tide, to change PE from a dreadfully obligatory subject to an eagerly anticipated one. By making PE inclusive, focused on personal and social development, and embedded in everyday life context, we are laying the groundwork for a generation of physically active, emotionally resilient, and socially responsible young people. With the purpose of changing our approach towards Physical Education, we can, indeed, reinvent the future.

Chapter 3. Unleashing the Power of Teamwork: Collaborative Learning in Sports

As we delve into the innovative terrain of Physical Education, we are immediately met with the force that is Teamwork. Not merely a tool to be used on the sports field, but a skill to be honed, exploited and celebrated, Teamwork holds power beyond our comprehension. Sports provide the perfect pitch to exercise this power, bridging gaps in social dynamics, building connections, and fostering a sense of responsibility and empathy among students. It's time to unravel the prowess that belongs to Teamwork, all while actively engaging students in sports.

3.1. The Role of Teamwork in Sport and Education

It's essential to value and understand the influential role of teamwork within the context of both sport and education. In the sporting realm, teamwork presents itself as the binding force, enabling teams to strategize, communicate, and drive towards their shared objective – victory. It can often be the defining factor between a good team and a great team, as synergy and coordination often trump individual skills.

In an educational context, the importance of teamwork extends far beyond the confines of the sports field. Collaboratively, students have been seen to grow, not only in their academic pursuits but as developing individuals. They gain essential social skills, empathy, and a collective understanding and responsibility. By integrating teamwork into sports education, we blend the worlds of personal development and athletic growth, creating a holistic and robust education structure.

3.2. Building the Foundation: Identifying Teamwork Elements

When we speak of teamwork in a broad sense, certain intrinsic elements emerge, which underpin the concept. These elements include communication, cooperation, respect, role clarity, and conflict resolution.

Communication is the lifeblood of any thriving team. A team that communicates efficiently navigates smoothly through obstacles, adapting and growing together.

Cooperation, the very essence of teamwork, is an indispensable asset. It encourages players to collaborate, value each other's strengths and compensate for their weaknesses.

Respect fosters a healthy and positive team environment. Respect for rules, coaches, team members, and competitors is of utmost importance in sports and beyond.

Role clarity maintains a balance and understanding between team members. When everyone knows and respects their role and responsibility, it reduces ambiguity and friction within the team.

Conflict resolution, an often overlooked aspect, is beneficial both on and off the field. By encouraging students to resolve their issues strategically and amicably, we equip them with an essential life skill.

3.3. The Process: Encouraging Collaborative Learning

The method of facilitation is crucial in encouraging a teamwork-focused approach in sports. Integrating small group activities or team-based tasks into regular practice can stimulate the development of teamwork.

Creating interdependencies within the team, using captains or leaders to guide smaller factions, and rotating these roles can help students understand both leadership and role clarity.

Building in-game scenarios that need collaboration and team strategizing can be a catalyst for developing the necessary skills. Regular reflection and feedback on team dynamics and interpersonal relationships also play a pivotal role in nurturing a teamwork-oriented environment.

3.4. The Impact: Benefits of Teamwork

The impact of focusing on teamwork resounds loudly in the domain of sports and reflects far beyond the field. It instills essential skill sets - negotiation, strategic planning, adaptive learning and more, in students, thereby setting them up for success in their futures.

In conclusion, the power of teamwork has the capacity to reform sports education. Collaborative learning in sports is not merely a teaching methodology but a transformative tool, capable of building healthier, more adaptive and socially equipped students. Through a persistent focus on teamwork and collaborative learning, we have the potential to create substantial benefits for our students' personal and athletic development. As we move forward in reimagining Physical Education, let's harness the power of teamwork to cultivate an environment of active and engaged learning.

Chapter 4. Advancing Beyond the Norm: Innovative PE Techniques for Active Learning

In the pathway of transforming conventional PE, it's essential to adopt a set of innovative tools and techniques. These serve to break down the walls of repetitive routines and instead look towards an inclusive, engaging, and effective learning environment.

4.1. Capitalising on Game-Based Learning

Game-based learning is one strategy that capitalises on children's natural affinity for games. Games promote active involvement, curiosity, and initiative, providing a viable platform for motivating students in otherwise daunting physical activities. Incorporating games into your curriculum allows the integration of problem-solving, cognitive development, and coordination, all while keeping learners engaged.

One example is 'Fitness Monopoly', modeled after the iconic board game. Each square signifies a different exercise, and students perform that exercise as they land on the respective squares. Regularly changing the activities in the squares fosters unpredictability and intrigue, keeping the game fresh.

4.2. Developing Individual Champions with Personal Goal Setting

Personal goal setting charts a pathway for children to continuously enhance their physical capabilities. As opposed to comparative objectives, which may demoralise less gifted students, each child pursues their individual fitness journey. This nurtures self-confidence and determination while ensuring constant progress. Encourage learners to set SMART (Specific, Measurable, Achievable, Relevant, Time-bound) goals, encapsulating both short-term and long-term objectives.

4.3. Leveraging Technology Integration

Virtual reality (VR) technology is one example of how tech can revolutionise PE. VR sporting platforms serve not only as an exciting new avenue for participation but also for heightening physical capabilities. From virtual soccer to boxing, these technologies inculcate a seamless blend of entertainment and comprehensive physical training.

Another is fitness tracking wearables. These devices, equipped with heart rate monitors, accelerometer, and GPS, provide real-time data – assisting students in understanding their bodies better and curating their fitness regimens.

4.4. Encouraging Collaborative Learning

Collaborative learning is an essential aspect of comprehensive development, fostering responsibility and cooperation among students. Cooperative games, obstacle courses designed for teams, and off-the-beat sports like dragon boat racing can spark a fun-filled team spirit. Once students work together towards a common goal, they realise the significance of unity and the power of mutual encouragement.

4.5. Learning through Outdoor Adventure Activities

Mother nature offers an exceptional gymnasium, and educators should capitalise on it. Outdoor adventure activities like hiking, rock climbing, or orienteering significantly bolster personal strengths and resilience while enhancing fitness levels. Similarly, they imbibe in children a sense of respect for the environment.

Independent navigation through orienteering, for instance, sparks independence and gives students a sense of achievement. Overcoming the hurdles of rock climbing instills confidence and determination.

4.6. Incorporating Mind-Body Disciplines

Bringing disciplines such as Yoga, Tai Chi, or Pilates into the fold can bridge the gap between physical education and mental wellbeing. These mind-body practices not only strengthen the body but also foster concentration, patience, relaxation, and self-awareness. Incorporating these practices can lay the foundations of mindful fitness, sparking a lifelong bond with fitness rooted at a deeper, more beneficial level.

4.7. Tailoring Student Fitness Plans

Every child is unique, with specific abilities and fitness levels. Therefore, adopting a one-size-fits-all approach could be counterproductive. Instead, tailored fitness plans for each student offer significant advantages. This strategy respects student uniqueness and involves catering to their individual strengths and working on their weaknesses.

Custom-fit plans can be built around the feedback loop - monitor, measure (using fitness assessment), review, and adjust. Through this dynamic process, the proposed fitness activities constantly evolve, maintaining relevance and fostering consistent progress.

Now more than ever, we need to be innovative in our approach to ensure that physical education serves its purpose - fostering lifetime fitness habits and overall well-being, all while keeping the process exciting and fulfilling. Taking physical education beyond the conventional, through intriguing and unconventional techniques, is fundamental in bringing about true, meaningful change. Together, let's promote a holistic learning environment that capitalises on student enthusiasm for an active, healthier future.

Chapter 5. Bridging the Rift: Encouraging Physical Fitness and Enjoyment

The rift between physical education and children's genuine enjoyment needs bridging. It isn't just about instilling fitness habits but also about fostering a lifelong love for activity, camaraderie, and the games themselves.

5.1. Reframing Perceptions: Making PE Fun

Perhaps one of the most significant challenges in this endeavor is reshaping how children perceive physical education. For too long, PE has carried the reputation of being a necessary yet dull and tedious part of the school curriculum. Long laps to run, monotone instructors, and dull exercises have been the bane of gym classes.

Yet, PE doesn't have to be this way. By harnessing the transformative power of games, teachers can reform the students' experience, making it less about rote exercises and more about the joy that comes with play. Incorporating elements such as teamwork can further help children view gym classes as more than just an individual physical exertion obligation but a collective, fun, character-building exercise.

5.2. The Magic of Gamification

Gamification relies upon incorporating game-like elements, such as point systems, competition, and rewards, to an otherwise possibly routine activity. In the context of physical education, this could translate into making each class more interactive and goal-oriented.

For instance, teachers could set up weekly challenges with rewards that act as incentives for children to participate, make an effort, and most importantly, enjoy the process. This could involve a variety of activities, whether it's building an obstacle course, hosting a mini Olympics, or running a dance-off. By offering a diverse range of activities, students will have the opportunity to play to their strengths, discover new passions, and stay engaged.

5.3. Teamwork: Encouraging Healthy Competition and Cooperation

Physical education also provides an excellent opportunity to teach students about teamwork. Many sports and games require cooperation among team members to achieve a common goal, whether it's scoring goals in soccer or maneuvering a basketball court.

Distinct from traditional teaching modes, PE classes emphasizing team sports can impart essential life skills such as empathy, cooperation, leadership, negotiation, and conflict resolution. It transforms PE from an individualistic endeavor into a cooperative learning experience, instilling in students the idea that "we are all in this together." This communal aspect can make physical education more enjoyable for many students.

5.4. Tailoring to Individual Needs: The Inclusivity Factor

While incorporating teamwork and competition can make physical education more engaging, it's equally important that these aspects don't become intimidations. There can be a fine line between healthy competition and an environment that unduly stresses performance and victory over enjoyment and participation.

It's essential that gym classes accommodate various capabilities and interests. Teachers should pay attention to the individual differences among students and tailor activities to their distinct needs. Small steps like these can help build an inclusive, fun, and motivating environment for physical education.

5.5. The Importance of a Playful Spirit

A playful spirit is key to fostering enjoyment in physical education. When students look forward to PE as a break from the regular day, they are more likely to be engaged and active. Teachers can nurture this spirit by ensuring that PE's atmosphere is encouraging, inclusive, and full of joy, rather than one of duty and obligation. Doing so will not only improve children's overall physical health but also their mental well-being.

5.6. The Role of Self-Improvement and Personal Bests

Another aspect to consider while bridging the rift between physical fitness and enjoyment is the focus on self-improvement and chasing personal bests, rather than benchmarking against others' performance. Gym classes that put a premium on personal growth rather than ranking tend to instill a healthy regard for fitness and enhance the enjoyment aspect. This shift in outlook opens up a promising avenue to promote a love for sport and a life-long commitment to remaining active.

The challenge comes down to creating a transformative shift - from a dreaded obligation to an anticipated refuge of fun, engagement and personal development. This reinvention of PE necessitates a carefully balanced mix of gamified elements, competition, cooperative experiences, an inclusive approach, and an encouraging atmosphere. That, indeed, is the key to bridging the rift between fitness and enjoyment in physical education.

Chapter 6. The Science Behind Active Learning in Physical Education

The paradigm of Physical Education is drastically shifting, from it being perceived merely as a playground pursuit to a structured discipline that stimulates cognitive and social development alongside physical health and well-being.

6.1. The Cognitive Engagement in Active Learning

The key differentiator of active learning is the cognitive engagement that it promotes. Instead of rote drills and practice, students are encouraged to explore, solve problems, and make decisions within the spectrum of Physical Education activities.

Neuroscience shows that active learning, compared to passive learning, leads to better memory retention and understanding of new concepts. To understand this, let's look at the process of learning from a neurological perspective. A new skill or knowledge forms a neural pathway in the brain. Each subsequent practice or drill strengthens this pathway. Active learning encourages the activation of these neural pathways more intensely, leading to better retention and consolidation of new information.

A study by Michigan State University indicated that children who are physically fit are likely to have better language skills, cognitive flexibility, and working memory, compared to their less fit peers.

6.2. Active Learning and Sports: A Symbiotic Relationship

Sports, by definition, require the practitioner to be active, not just physically, but also mentally. The brain and body work in synergy, as one understands the rules of the game, develops game strategies, or learns to predict and react to opponents' moves.

Football, for example, involves understanding the rules, coordinating with team members, discerning the other team's dynamics, and executing strategic actions. This demands mental acuity and promotes cognitive fitness - enhancing memory, attention, creativity, and problem-solving abilities.

Sports also teach vital life skills such as discipline, teamwork, resilience, and leadership. Thus, embedding active learning into sports transforms Physical Education into a holistic learning experience that transcends mere physical activity.

6.3. Active Learning and Physical Fitness

Active learning not only fosters cognitive abilities and life skills but also plays a crucial role in instilling physical fitness. Incorporating active learning in Physical Education has been seen to increase students' vigilance in maintaining a healthy lifestyle.

Active learning empowers students to understand the importance of physical activity, the role of nutrition in fitness, and the need for a disciplined routine, making the lessons durable beyond the sports field. This proactive, immersed, and aware approach to health and fitness is a radical shift from the short-term, goal-oriented perspective that traditional fitness training espouses.

6.4. Measuring Outcomes of Active Learning in Physical Education

The outcomes of active learning in Physical Education can be evaluated considering three domains: physical, cognitive, and social.

Physical outcomes include measurable improvements in one's aerobic capacity, muscle strength, balance, physical activity levels, and technical sport skills.

The cognitive domain explores how sports-based active learning impacts students' academic performance, especially in areas requiring executive functions, subsequent attention abilities, memory, and knowledge retention.

Social outcomes include improved cooperation, empathy, negotiation skills, and team spirit. They also incorporate a better understanding of sports ethics, leadership, resilience, and discipline.

6.5. Conclusion: The Future of Physical Education

Active learning brings a refreshing, engaging, and holistic approach to Physical Education, enriching the student's physical, cognitive, and social skills. This comprehensive model of learning redefines Physical Education, positioning it beyond the traditional constructs of fitness training. It recreates Physical Education as a dynamic spectrum, where fitness training, cognition, and social interaction intersect, furthering the overall development of the individual.

Through the adoption of active learning, Physical Education is stepping into a future where every student is an engaged participant, keen to explore, understand, and grow. As the science supporting active learning solidifies, it is becoming increasingly clear that the benefits are far-reaching, paving the way for a healthier, intellectually stimulated, and socially aware generation.

Chapter 7. Revitalizing Curriculum: Key Strategies for Engagement and Participation

The heart of any effective Physical Education program lies in an engaging and inclusive curriculum. It's time to break away from repetitive routines and launch an innovative approach, one that revolves around active and collaborative learning techniques to ignite a passion for sports and fitness in students.

7.1. The Power behind Purposeful Play

General gym class activities tend to be met with begrudging participation or lack thereof. Why? Because they often lack purpose in the eyes of the students. To conquer this, we must introduce the concept of 'Purposeful Play.' This integrates learning objectives with fun physical activities, making the education process enjoyable and effective. For instance, playing tag can be seen as a simple, entertaining game, but it can concurrently teach students about teamwork, strategy, and agility.

Purposeful play utilizes games and sports where students can learn and apply skills in real-time, promoting higher retention. This, coupled with its fun element, encourages maximum participation, driving the overall success of the Physical Education program.

7.2. Inspiring Autonomy through Personal Goals

While team sports and games teach essential collaborative skills, personal fitness goals can inspire individual commitment and autonomy. This approach allows children to focus on their personal fitness development at a pace that suits them and achieve measurable, realistic goals.

Personal goals provide strong motivation for the student, as they are directly linked to their improvement. Regular tracking of their progress and continuous feedback would ensure that they are actively engaged and participating, contributing to their feeling of accomplishment.

7.3. Technology Integration

Every student today is a digital native. We can tap into their interest in technology to foster fitness goals. Gadgets like fitness trackers can instantly appeal to their penchant for technology while enabling them to monitor their vital statistics and progress in real-time.

Physical Education programs can integrate with health and fitness apps to provide a personalized learning experience. Simple additions like creating leaderboards or rewards for students who achieve their goals can increase participation and produce a competitive, productive classroom environment.

7.4. Differentiated Instruction

One size does not fit all, especially in Physical Education. While some students might thrive in fast-paced sports, others might prefer slower, methodological activities. Understanding these differences and implementing differentiated instruction is a key strategy towards fostering engagement and promoting participation.

Differentiated instruction organizes activities based on students' abilities, interests, and learning preferences. This ensures every learner can participate and contribute, promoting inclusive physical education. Regular assessments can help teachers differentiate instruction effectively based on students' needs, thus ensuring continued engagement.

7.5. Active Learning

Traditional physical education focuses on teaching techniques and rules often without a proper context, disconnecting students from real application. Active learning strategies, on the other hand, place the student at the center of the learning process.

Students learn by doing, discovering, and solving problems, which ensures they are active participants, not passive recipients. Activities like Adventure Sports or Outdoor Education, where they learn navigational skills, tend to stimulate their cognitive skills and arouse curiosity, thus promoting active participation.

7.6. Cultivating Sportsmanship and Healthy Competition

An often overlooked aspect of Physical Education - sportsmanship and fair play - can be instrumental in enhancing student engagement. Students should be taught to compete, but also to respect opponents, the rules of the game, and to appreciate playing for the sake of enjoyment itself.

By encouraging sportsmanship, we cultivate an environment of respect and admiration among students. This encourages them to participate actively without the fear of failure, knowing they are part of an accepting, constructive community.

In conclusion, these strategies are by no means exhaustive but usher in a fresh approach to the traditional models of Physical Education. They aim at not only sustaining interest and active participation in PE but also at equipping students with skills and knowledge that extend beyond the boundaries of the gymnasium.

Revamping the curriculum considering these strategies can indeed have a transformative impact, creating an active, engaged, and enthusiastic learning culture. Change begins with each one of us - let us play our part in revitalizing Physical Education and redefine it as an enlightening and empowering journey for every student.

Chapter 8. Psychology Meets Physical Education: Understanding Student Motivation

Physical Education (PE) is much more than sets of movements or exercises. It's a spectrum of activities that foster physical health, but alongside, they also shape the cognitive abilities of students, enhancing their understanding of discipline, sportsmanship, teamwork, and ultimately self-efficacy. To understand how psychological factors influence students' motivation towards PE, we need to delve deep into the intertwined relationship between psychology and physical education.

8.1. Intrinsic and Extrinsic Motivation

Before we explore the role of psychology in PE, it's essential to acknowledge two fundamental types of motivation, intrinsic and extrinsic. Intrinsic motivation arises from within the individual. It's driven by personal satisfaction or the inherent joy of performing a task. Extrinsic motivation, on the other hand, is fueled by external rewards such as accolades, tokens, or commendations.

The theory of **Self-Determination** is pivotal to understanding these forms of motivation. Proposed by psychologists Deci and Ryan, it emphasizes that individuals are more motivated when they feel autonomy, competence, and relatedness. In PE, enhancing these elements can significantly influence students' motivation.

8.2. Translating Psychological Theories to Physical Education

The **Goal Orientation Theory** suggests people are either task-oriented or ego-oriented. Task-oriented individuals see effort as a way to mastery and derive satisfaction from personal improvement. On the other hand, ego-oriented individuals gauge their ability in comparison with others, investing effort only if they believe they can showcase superior performance.

PE instructors can harness this theory by promoting task orientation, emphasizing personal growth and effort, rather than just focusing on winning.

Attribution Theory highlights how individuals interpret and understand their successes and failures. Some kids attribute their success to external factors like luck and failure to a lack of ability. It's critical to shift this mindset, teaching students that consistent effort and effective strategies lead to successful outcomes in physical activities.

8.3. Promoting Positive Affirmations in PE Classes

Positive affirmations have a profound impact on boosting self-confidence and motivation. Phrases like "I can do this" or "I am getting better with each step" can notably affect students' approach towards physical activities. Simplifying complex movements into smaller, achievable parts can help students believe in their ability to perform challenging tasks.

8.4. Understanding Anxiety in PE

Anxiety and fear of judgment often deter students from participating actively in PE classes. Social anxiety, performance anxiety, and fear of injury are some common forms of anxiety experienced. Addressing these fears and adopting an empathetic approach can promote a positive learning environment where students feel comfortable taking risks and making mistakes.

8.5. Challenges of Modern Technology

We are living in a digital world, where screen time is increasing exponentially. Video games, social media, and online entertainment channels are making kids less active, posing significant challenges to PE. Strategies used in these digital spaces, such as offering levels of challenge and opportunities for control and choices, can be applied effectively within PE curriculum to ignite students' interest and engagement.

8.6. Evaluation as Motivation

Evaluation in PE often creates a stressful environment for students. If it's about winning and losing, assessment can become a demotivating factor. However, constructive feedback focusing on personal improvement can turn evaluation into a motivational tool. The essence should lie in "competence" rather than "competition."

8.7. Building a Collaborative Environment

Collaborative learning in PE can foster a sense of relatedness, building stronger relationships among students. Group activities and team sports teach students values of respect, trust, and understanding different perspectives, instilling in them essential life skills and boosting their motivation towards PE.

To conclude, understanding student motivation in PE isn't a linear process. It's a multi-dimensional phenomenon, involving intricate psychological theories to pragmatic teaching strategies. A sound comprehension of these aspects will work wonders in reinventing PE, making it an anticipated class rather than an obligation, leading to healthier, happier, and holistically developed students.

Chapter 9. Boosting Cognitive Performance Through Physical Education: The Mind-Body Connection

On a fundamental level, we know a sound body breeds a sound mind. The linkage between physical fitness and cognitive prowess is not just rhetoric; there's a wealth of scientific evidence to prove this claim. Over the last few years, we have seen a revival of interest in exploring the mind-body connection, and how to harness it to promote holistic development.

9.1. Taking a Cue from Neuroscience

Neuroscience has long been interested in the ways that physical education (PE) can enhance cognitive functioning. A surge of brain-derived neurotrophic factor (BDNF) - a protein that supports the survival of existing neurons and encourages the creation and growth of new neurons and synapses - is noticed when we exert ourselves physically.

Aerobic exercises like running, swimming, or even a brisk walk, can stimulate the production of this brain-building protein. This process is crucial in cognitive areas such as memory consolidation, learning, and higher thinking. These insights initiate an exciting dialogue about the possibilities of boosting cognitive performance through physical education.

9.2. Making the Most of Motor Skills

Another suggestion on how physical education can enhance cognitive performance comes from the study of motor skills. Motor learning, which requires the brain to coordinate with the body to perform complex movements, can be developed in a physical education setting. Whether it's throwing a ball, balancing on a beam, or running a track, physical activities offer ample opportunity for enhancing and honing motor skills.

Understanding motor learning can help students improve their problem-solving abilities and executive function, which involves skills like organization, planning, and executing tasks. A systematized sports process isn't just physical, but cognitive, requiring one to process and decide on the best course of action.

9.3. Facilitating Learning through Exercise

Educationists worldwide are beginning to realize the correlation between exercise and improved learning outcomes. The vast array of physical activities, involving a combination of cardio, strength, flexibility, and agility, can have a remarkable impact on cognitive development.

The physical exertion that comes from exercise prompts the brain to release chemicals such as dopamine and norepinephrine, which promote mood improvement, attention, and memory. These neurochemical changes can facilitate an environment conducive to learning.

9.4. Unleashing the Potential of Mindful Movement

Mindful movement practices, like yoga or tai chi, bring added dimensions of relaxation, concentration, and self-awareness. These activities are not only beneficial for physical health but also support stress management and emotional resilience - factors critical for effective learning.

Participants focused on their breath, posture, and specific movement during a yoga sequence, enabling them to stay engaged and directed towards the task at hand. This focus may lead to improved concentration, attention span, and self-discipline, that are all transferable to academic tasks.

9.5. A Healthy Body Equals a Healthy Brain

A physically fit student is not merely healthier; they're more attuned to their cognitive abilities. The connection between physical fitness and cognitive performance isn't new, but it's been under-emphasized in traditional gym class structures.

By focusing on the aspects of physical education that enhance cognitive functioning, such as aerobic exercises, complex motor skills learning, regular exercise regimes, and mindfulness activities, we can build a generation equipped with not just knowledge but cognitive fitness. Physical education effectively becomes a tool for teaching students that a healthy body does indeed lead to a healthy brain, thereby encouraging lifelong habits of regular physical activity and mental acuity.

In the end, it's not about creating superstar athletes but encouraging students to participate, engage, and understand the essential mind-body correlation. It's not just about victory over others, but a victory over one's self. Boosting cognitive performance through physical education becomes a reality when students make those connections - and that's a way of learning that will serve them throughout their lives.

Chapter 10. Measuring Success: Assessment Techniques in the Active Learning Model

In the realm of Physical Education, success isn't just determined by how fast a student can run a lap or how high they can jump. In an active learning model, assessing success goes beyond mere physical prowess and delves into aspects of teamwork, strategic thinking, persistence, and personal growth. To measure success appropriately, an array of innovative and contextually appropriate assessment techniques need to be employed.

10.1. The Paradigm Shift: From Performative to Holistic Assessment

Assessing success in Physical Education goes beyond measuring physical attributes like strength and agility. It delves into a well-rounded approach, taking into account the cognitive, effective, and behavioral aspects linked to the learning objectives. This shift calls for assessment techniques that focus on the student's understanding, strategic thinking, and consistent performance over time.

In the past, assessment was heavily centered on skills demonstration, occasional fitness tests, and infrequent games performance. These traditional methods often failed to take holistic development into account, focusing on physical development while sidelining the important aspects of cognitive, psychomotor, and affective learning.

Now, the spotlight is on factors such as understanding the rules of the game, strategizing action plans, social skills, and personal development. This approach paves the way to assess students more effectively and fairly, painting a complete picture of their progress in the subject.

10.2. Assessment Techniques in the Active Learning Model

To make the process of assessing holistic learning effective, we're introducing innovative and contextually appropriate assessment techniques.

1. Performance-based Assessment: Evaluates a student's ability to execute a specific skill or tactic. This goes beyond physical prowess and includes strategic thinking and game sense. These assessments can be formative (giving ongoing feedback) or summative (assessing the student's performance at the end of an instructional unit).

2. Observation and Anecdotal Notes: Teachers keep an eye on students during class and make notes on their performance. This informal, day-to-day method helps in tracking individual progress over time.

3. Portfolio Assessment: A physical or digital collection of a student's work and performances. These archives can include videos of games, personal reflections, written assignments, self-assessment scores, and peer-assessment feedback.

4. Interviews and Conferences: One-to-one interactions between the teacher and student to discuss progress, challenges, strategies, and goals.

5. Journals and Logs: Students maintain records of their activities, experiences, thoughts, and reflections. These can contain self-evaluation notes, indicating what the students think they're doing well and where they need to improve.

6. Self and Peer Assessment: Students evaluate their own and their

peers' performances. This technique fosters a sense of personal responsibility and encourages teamwork.

7. Rubrics: These are scoring guides used to evaluate the quality of students' tasks or performances. They consist of criteria that reflect the learning objectives, along with descriptors to define the different levels of proficiency.

10.3. The Importance of Rubrics in Assessment

Rubrics are crucial tools in the assessment process. They provide a structured framework which helps students understand what is expected of them, guides educators in evaluating achievements, and ensures the assessments' efficacy and fairness.

Creating a good rubric starts with clearly defined learning objectives. Once these are in place, the different criteria should be linked to these objectives, defining what an excellent, good, fair, or poor performance looks like for each. Rubrics can be adapted for various games, sports activities, cognitive tasks, and behaviour assessments.

Properly used, rubrics provide the students with clarity about their goals, helping them understand what is expected and how to grow and improve. For teachers, rubrics make the assessment process more efficient and accurate, providing a consistent framework by which to measure every student's progress.

10.4. The Role of Formative Assessment and Feedback

In the world of active learning, formative assessments play a critical role. These ongoing assessments provide immediate feedback to students, helping them identify their strengths and areas that need improvement. Armed with this information, students can tweak their strategies, apply new techniques, or practice certain skills. For teachers, formative assessments offer insights into student comprehension, informing their teaching methods and strategies.

Feedback is integral to formative assessments. Constructive feedback should provide students with specific information on their performance, focus on positive achievements as well as areas that need improvement, and offer suggestions on how to make progress. Engaging students in the feedback process, for example by asking them to self-assess their work or evaluate their peers, helps develop critical thinking and judgment skills.

10.5. Conclusion: Towards a Comprehensive Assessment System

Embedding assessments in every step of active learning makes the process integral to teaching and learning in Physical Education. These innovative and context-sensitive assessment techniques make the process more comprehensive and holistic, moving us away from a merely performative measurement of success.

Bringing these techniques together presents us with a comprehensive assessment system that challenges one-dimensional views of success in PE, honoring the multifaceted nature of physical, cognitive and socio-emotional growth. Each component — from performance-based assessments to the use of rubrics — contributes to a more accurate picture of each student's development, leading to a more conducive learning environment that empowers, enlightens, and enlivens every learner.

This is the key to transforming the way we teach and learn Physical Education, making every child look forward to each PE class with enthusiasm and excitement. Stepping into this new wave of assessment is stepping into the future of Physical Education. As educators, let's embrace this shift and witness the empowering transformation of our students as they enjoy and learn from the vibrant world of Physical Education.

Chapter 11. Charting the Future: Policy Recommendations for a Reinvented PE

In anticipation of a transformative shift in Physical Education policy and delivery, it's important to be armed with an arsenal of innovative, well-founded, and student-friendly policy recommendations. These directions not only reinvent the PE experience but also seek to inspire students to actively invest in their fitness journey.

11.1. The Holistic Approach

A holistic approach to PE includes physical, cognitive, and emotional development. This concept understands that a child's engagement in physical activity is just as essential for their mental and emotional growth.

The government should aim to implement a policy that ensures every school incorporates a holistic PE curriculum. Such a curriculum should emphasize not just the physical aspect, but also sportsmanship, team building, resilience, and self-esteem. It should also provide opportunities for students to explore various recreational activities beyond traditional competitive sports, like yoga, dance, outdoor adventures, and more.

11.2. Versatility is the Key

If we aim to captivate the diverse interests of all students, PE classes should offer a variety of activities. The policy must push for flexible and adjustable curriculums, where student voices are heard, and their preferences respected. This diversification encourages students to step out of their comfort zones, try new things without fear, and possibly discover new passions along the way.

11.3. Technological Integration

Today's children are digital natives; they have grown up in a technology-rich environment. Leveraging this will help make PE attractive and relevant to them. Policymakers should advocate for the integration of technology in PE. This may involve fitness trackers, virtual reality sports simulations, online fitness challenges— the possibilities are endless. Use of technology can make learning fun, provide immediate feedback, and allow individualized progression.

11.4. Teacher Training and Development

We cannot expect to revolutionize PE without focusing on the educational pillars - the teachers. Investing in ongoing professional development for PE educators is indispensable. Such training should focus not only on teaching various sports and activities but also on fostering an inclusive, supportive, and enjoyable learning environment. The policies should further aim to promote a forum for teachers to exchange ideas and share their best practices.

11.5. Inclusive Learning Environments

PE environments should celebrate diversity and inclusivity. Thus, it's crucial that policymakers underline the need for adapting activities to various fitness levels, abilities, and interests, thereby ensuring no student is left behind. Furthermore, inclusive PE guidelines could foster confidence, empathy, and mutual respect among students.

11.6. Healthy Competition

While encouraging competitiveness in sports is important, it's equally necessary not to discourage those who are naturally less competitive. Policymakers should ensure PE policies reflect this balance, promoting competitiveness while simultaneously focusing on effort, growth, progress, and personal achievements.

11.7. Regular Evaluation and Feedback

Policies that insist on regular assessments not only of physical abilities but of attitudes, team spirit, and sportsmanship are integral to the holistic growth ethos. Feedback should aim to encourage the students, fuel their motivation, and guide them towards personal development.

11.8. Parental Involvement

Engaging parents in their child's PE journey can be incredibly beneficial. Policymakers should consider policies to encourage school-home communication regarding the child's progress. This could include parents being informed about their child's fitness levels and how they can support them at home.

11.9. Encouraging Extra-Curricular Physical Activities

The scope of PE must extend beyond the school hours. Encouragement of extra-curricular physical activities like sports clubs, interschool competitions, or community runs, can foster a lifelong love for fitness.

11.10. Start Early

Exploring physical exercise must begin at a young age. Implementing PE right from the kindergarten phase can foster in children an early love and understanding of fitness, teamwork, and sportsmanship.

With these dynamic policy recommendations, we have the potential to revolutionize PE for the better. By adopting these, we can elevate the joy of movement to its rightful place, engaging hearts and minds and setting up our future generations for a lifetime of physical and emotional health.